WHIPPLE'S DISEASE

UNDERSTANDING THE HEALING PROCESS

OF WHIPPLE'S DISEASE

DR. KATE .P

Contents

CHAPTER ONE

INTRODUCTION

A rare bacterial infection, whipple's disease typically affects the gastrointestinal tract. Whipple's illness affects how well food breaks down, including fats and carbs, and how well your body absorbs nutrients, all of which can cause problems with regular digestion.

The brain, heart, joints, and eyes are among the other organs that can become infected by Whipple's illness.

Inappropriate care can make Whipple's disease dangerous or even deadly. Whipple's illness can, however, be treated with an antibiotic course.

Symptoms

Typical indications and symptoms

Whipple's disease frequently presents with gastrointestinal signs and symptoms, which can include:

The diarrhea

cramps and pain in the abdomen that could get worse after eating

Loss of weight linked to nutritional malabsorption

The following are some common indications and symptoms of Whipple's disease:

swollen joints, especially in your wrists, ankles, and knees

Weary

Deficiency

Anemia

less typical indications and symptoms

Signs and symptoms of Whipple's illness might occasionally include:

High temperature

Cough

swollen lymph nodes

Hyperpigmentation, or darkening of the skin, in sun-exposed areas and around scars chest ache

enlarged spleen

Among the neurological symptoms and indicators are:

walking challenges

impairment of vision, including inability to control eye motions

Convulsions

Perplexity

loss of memory

Most patients with this disease experience a gradual onset of symptoms over many years. Certain symptoms, such weight loss and joint discomfort, can appear years before the gastrointestinal symptoms that trigger a diagnosis.

When to visit a physician

Whipple's illness is usually curable but has the potential to be fatal. If you have strange symptoms or indicators, including unexplained weight loss or joint pain, get in touch with your doctor. Tests might be conducted by your doctor to identify the source of your symptoms.

Inform your physician if, after having therapy and a diagnosis of infection, your symptoms don't go better. Antibiotic therapy may not always work because the bacteria have developed resistance to the specific medication you are taking. Because the condition can return, it's critical to keep an eye out for any resurgence of symptoms.

Reasons

The bacterium Tropheryma whipplei is the source of Whipple's illness. This bacterium first causes minor lesions in the intestinal wall of your small intestine's mucosal lining. The tiny, hair-like projections (villi) that line the small intestine are also harmed by the bacteria. The infection may eventually spread to other body parts.

We don't know a lot about the bacteria. Scientists are not exactly sure where it originates from or how it is transmitted to humans, despite the fact that it appears to be easily found in the environment. Not all carriers of the bacteria go on to get sick. According to some experts, individuals who have the illness might be more vulnerable to contracting the bacterium when exposed to it due to a genetic abnormality in their immune system response.

Whipple's illness is incredibly rare.

RISK ELEMENTS

The bacterium that causes Whipple's disease is so poorly understood that risk factors for the illness are unclear. Reports currently available suggest that it is more likely to impact:

Men

Individuals between the ages of 40 and 60

White people in Europe and North America

COMMITMENTS

The tiny projections (villi) that resemble hairs on the walls of the small intestine aid in the body's absorption of nutrients. Villi damage from Whipple's illness reduces the body's ability to absorb nutrients. People with Whipple's illness frequently experience nutritional deficits, which can cause weakness, exhaustion, weight loss, and joint discomfort.

Whipple's illness is a degenerative condition that can be lethal. Despite the infection's rarity, deaths linked to it are still being documented;

this is mostly because of delayed diagnosis and treatment. The central nervous system becomes infected and can sustain irreversible damage, which frequently results in death.

Getting Ready for Your Consultation

See your physician as soon as possible if you exhibit symptoms that are typical of Whipple's disease. Whipple's illness is uncommon, and diagnosing it can be challenging because its symptoms and indications often mimic those of other, more prevalent conditions. It is frequently diagnosed in its latter stages as a result. On the other hand, the chance of major health consequences from not treating the illness is decreased with an early diagnosis.

CHAPTER TWO

Based on the symptoms you're experiencing, your doctor may recommend you to a specialist in digestive illnesses or to another medical professional if the diagnosis is unclear.

Here are some details to help you prepare for your visit and understand what to anticipate from your physician.

Information to obtain beforehand

Put your symptoms in writing, together with the time you first noticed them and any changes or worsening over time.

Put all of your important medical information in writing, including the names of all the drugs, vitamins, and supplements you are taking and any additional conditions you have been diagnosed with.

Important details about you, such as any recent changes or stresses in your life, should be put in writing. Digestive symptoms and indicators may be related to these causes.

If you can, bring a friend or member of your family. It's possible that someone with you will recall something you overlooked or forgot.

Prepare a list of inquiries for your physician. To maximize your time with your doctor, prepare your list of questions ahead of time.

Typical Whipple's disease signs and symptoms include the following, so be sure to ask your doctor these essential questions:

What is my condition's most likely cause?

Exist any further reasons why my illness might exist?

Which tests for diagnosis do I require?

Which course of treatment would you suggest?

I also suffer from other health issues. How can I oversee them collectively?

How quickly do you think my treatment will alleviate my symptoms?

How long will I have to take these drugs?

Are complications from this illness a possibility for me?

Can I expect a recurrence?

How often must you come visit me for observation?

Should I alter my diet?

Do I need to take any dietary supplements?

Can I alter my lifestyle in any way to assist manage or lessen my symptoms?

Please feel free to ask any other questions you may have.

When examining you for a potential case of Whipple's illness, your physician may inquire about the following:

What symptoms do you have, and when did you first notice them?

Have you had worsening symptoms over time?

Do your symptoms usually get worse right after eating?

Have you dropped a few pounds on your own?

Do you have joint pain?

Do you feel worn out or weak?

Do you cough or are you having trouble breathing?

Have you started to experience memory loss or confusion?

Have you experienced eyesight or eye issues?

Has anyone you know recently experienced comparable symptoms or signs?

Have you received a diagnosis for any additional illnesses, such as food allergies?

Do you have a family history of colon cancer or intestinal disorders?

Which prescription and over-the-counter drugs, vitamins, herbal remedies, and supplements do you now take?

Do you have any pharmaceutical allergies?

In order to diagnose Whipple's illness, the following tests are usually performed:

physical examination. During a physical examination, your doctor will probably start by checking for symptoms and indicators that point to the existence of this ailment, such as stomach pain and skin darkening, especially on areas of your body that have been exposed to the sun.

autopsy. A biopsy, which involves removing a sample usually from the small intestine lining, is a crucial step in the diagnosis of Whipple's illness. Your doctor usually does an upper endoscopy to accomplish this. A narrow, flexible scope is used for the procedure, and it goes through your mouth, neck, esophagus, stomach, and small intestine. Your doctor can take biopsies and observe your digestive tract thanks to the scope.

Tissue samples are taken from several intestinal locations during the process. The tissue is inspected under a microscope to check for the presence of bacteria that cause disease, their lesions, and Tropheryma whipplei bacteria in particular. In the event that small intestine biopsies are inconclusive, your physician may biopsy an enlarged lymph node or order additional tests.

Some medical institutes offer a polymerase chain reaction test that uses DNA to identify

Tropheryma whipplei bacteria in biopsy specimens or spinal fluid samples.

blood examinations. Additionally, your physician can prescribe blood tests, such a complete blood count. Certain disorders linked to Whipple's illness can be identified by blood testing, especially low albumin (a protein in the blood) and anemia (a decrease in red blood cell count).

MEDICATIONS AND SUBTLES

Antibiotics are used in combination or alone to treat Whipple's disease because they can eradicate the bacterium that is causing the illness.

The goal of the long-term, usually one or two-year treatment is to eradicate the germs. However, symptom relief usually occurs considerably more quickly, frequently in the first week or two. After taking antibiotics for the whole time, the majority of patients who do not have any issues with their brain or neurological system recover fully.

When doctors choose antibiotics, they frequently go for those that not only treat digestive tract infections but also penetrate the blood-brain barrier, which is a layer of tissue surrounding the brain, to get rid of germs that might have gotten into the brain and central nervous system.

Your doctor will need to keep an eye on your condition to make sure that resistance to the antibiotics develops because of the prolonged usage of these medications. Your doctor may decide to switch your antibiotics if you relapse while receiving treatment.

Handling of typical cases

Therapy for Whipple's illness often starts with intravenous (IV) ceftriaxone (Rocephin) for 14 days. You will probably be prescribed an oral course of sulfamethoxazole-trimethoprim, or SMX-TMP (Bactrim, Septra), for one to two years after that initial therapy. A recurrence could result from stopping antibiotic treatment too soon.

Ceftriaxone with SMX-TMP may cause mild diarrhea, nausea, and vomiting as side effects.

In the event that you exhibit neurologic symptoms, you can be prescribed oral doxycycline (Vibramycin) along with hydroxychloroquine (Plaquenil), an antimalarial medication, for a duration of 12 to 18 months. Long-term antibiotics like TMP-SMX, which can penetrate the brain and cerebrospinal fluid, will also be administered to you.

Doxycycline adverse effects include appetite loss, nausea, vomiting, and photosensitivity. Hydrychloroquine may result in headaches, dizziness, diarrhea, and an appetite loss.

Alleviation of symptoms

When you begin antibiotic treatment, your symptoms should get better in one to two weeks and go away completely in approximately a month.

However, even when your symptoms get better rapidly, additional lab work could show that the bacteria is still present two or more years after you start taking antibiotics. Your doctor will use follow-up tests to help you decide when to stop taking antibiotics. Frequent monitoring can also reveal the emergence of treatment resistance, which is frequently manifested as a failure to experience symptom alleviation.

Whipple's disease might return even after treatment is effective. Regular checks are frequently advised by doctors. In the event that a recurrence has occurred, you will require more antibiotic medication.

Consuming dietary supplements

Whipple's disease patients have problems absorbing nutrients, so your doctor could advise taking vitamin and mineral supplements to make sure you're getting enough nutrients. Your body could need more calcium, iron, magnesium, folic acid, vitamin D, and other nutrients.

THE END